RHEUMA

William Gee is a poet and writer based in East London. His work often focuses on chronic illness, trauma, and the intersectionality between the two. His work has received a Bare Fiction prize for poetry, and a Troubadour Prize, and has appeared in *Bare Fiction*, *Rising*, *Roulade*, *Proletarian Poetry* and on the Troubadour Prize website.

Rheuma

Published by Bad Betty Press in 2020
www.badbettypress.com

Cover design by Amy Acre

Printed and bound in the United Kingdom

A CIP record of this book is available from the British Library.

ISBN: 978-1-913268-10-7

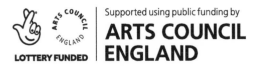

Supported using public funding by
ARTS COUNCIL ENGLAND
LOTTERY FUNDED

Rheuma

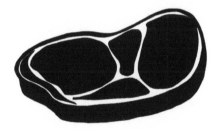

PRESS

Rheuma

For Lara

Contents

tomorrow my brother died

and any of the last words I might say to him will be expected when it happened
he was getting on a plane or tying his laces between parked cars not looking
when I am mouthing that I love him always even when I'm turning out the insides of my pockets
my shoulders making nothing of my neck my brother is dead my brother is dead my brother
wants to go out for lunch but he'll die instead in the photographs he will send me
he dies when I sleep in till eleven when I turn on my xbox and when I think of him
he is dying when I forget to brush my teeth and he's dead when I don't he's thrown himself
into the tube he's black coffee gone cold in the hand in each second he must think
his phone is not working

dead/hotdogs

your father is/was(sorry)/will be an accomplished lover
by which I mean he has loved was loving will love again
by which time I am already ruined   as skin after e45
soft or exemplary or the smell of hospitals
as do you remember your mum   yes as motorola razr
as twelve missed calls   as tell your mum   if you're reading this

      mum I will always love you

manage your expectations

breathe but not too much you're about to mistake your stomach
for your lungs swallow until your gut is breathing
this is the part where you start to feel sick your insides threatening
mate are you ok your redness is not only internal your face an embarrassment
of cheeks and throat and isn't it that life is one day after another or
is it your jeans needing washing your mind stupidly alight
your body unsuitable for the storage of its lunch

something manageable

is when I love people I drown them
I put them in planes and I take away their earth
and when they come back down it's easy you touch me
your hands survive my body and I love you for that

self talk

put your hands in your pockets and fold your shoulders in
so it looks like they're playing pinball with your head
smile even though you don't have any reason to smile
you just want to look normal and normal people smile
when they're walking down the street as if they're watching
comfy sitcoms in their heads or warming up
for when someone beautiful walks by

if you wipe your eyes with the cuff of your sleeve
  the tears you're blaming
    on the wind
won't run

if you don't someone might ask
  if you're ok

young man,

you are an expert in having lives to waste and how are we to love you like that
your body lacking in the confidence of your bedroom your body only faking
threedimensional separate from its own politics incapable of sending its meats
to the right places of unsending its acids and instead how hard
are you willing to work to get away from yourself young man take all
your beauty out from your natwest student account your beauty is modest as a box
room your beauty is always hungry in the same coat too small to be saved I'm sorry
come back when your body is its most successful factory when you've died
at all the punctured versions of yourself

please my pain

has been drinking is my literal ▮▮▮▮ threatening to turn on her back
in her sleep and years ago and then again I am keeping her door open
and it's painful when a promise goes on breaking in the long unbeautiful
morning always waking always coffee permaweak muscles
locked like a bad dog all teeth all stop please neverbad ▮▮▮▮
bad nights for you no sleep until and then
   soft beds
       lifetime of feathers
oh
  wrap up
 your working body

something manageable

is leaving the house is my stomach upwards my pain making holes
in the walls of my mouth is literal acid if I want to do anything

literally it's all the fingers

withoutpermissiontoholdme
   like that   my body
became everything and after (I'm sorry) my intimacy
there is room between us literally don't sleep because of it
   manage not to think of it except often
when my days end on the bus so close I belong
to whoever is pressed against my leg I'm
   twenty three now and still I keep my head blank
in case when accidentally my hand is touched
  greencarpetbedroomfloor
and all my boy memories
   lie down

  dontlookmybody
   isnotgood

something manageable

is keeping secrets is teeth in your stomach

damaged/good

when I was twelve I started to practice packing my whole body
inside my head if my mouth was shut I'd fit in and now
even when I'm talking I can taste myself I used to throw up
and after no one could look at me in the mornings when I shone
with sweat with sleeplessness a hand slipped in my boyhood
happened only once I lost control let's never talk about it

my ▮ ribs

and sometimes I stand in front of buses knowing they'll never hit
they get close and my body stops them don't even need to scream just my being
there is enough makes impact impossible before we even got out the door the world
was hitting my ▮ and however I threw my body it didn't stop and doesn't
it make sense now by the time my ▮ is protecting his ribs we're going to new york
and the whole way he is beautiful his side all blue all fists forgiven imagine every time
a hand is raised you have to brace for impact or walk into it

oh soul

you are indeed what carries on
insufferable to form you are all of autumn
& most of clapton square has come
down I am kicking my big shoes
through its going leaves &
my hair looks wrong
        my obvious stomach
oh baby
     I baby my body into this
particular shape
when you leave I am one
sad question mark
curled up around my knees
on this bench I want to let go
     of what's left
crushing yellow
handful of sunsets
my big
     impossible self

to the people I work with

are you embarrassed yet
I am sitting out the morning
& you know it I am bathroom missing
& not so many feet away
you switch your radio on and I
spilling my guts could kiss you till your lips melt
on my knees my life seems pretty
low trapped almost always between living
& cubical my body breaking its own confidence
you know the way I hold myself
& when finally I am at my desk
forgive me put your hand on my still
dripping hand
move me like I am working

mother, like me

in pain the cake is unbelievable
my mouth goes sweetly quiet and you hold me
like nothing can't be swallowed I let this happen
put my pain down for a second my stomach so ugly heavy
my broken oesophageal valve all fat and acid
my mixed up insides
I'm sorry mum   let me keep this mouth-
ful forever let nothing come up
let me keep this mouth
    full all I can taste is love I am soaked
in it I am the wringing out of pain
I am always
    impossibly
 sponge

nonrestorative sleep

& sometimes this sick can be beautiful
I suck in air wake up all stomach all breath

        can I tell you
how each minute of dead quiet morning
will taste of course I can I have
almost all night awake in my lungs
I am a space I practice expanding
often I make rooms I fill them up
with pain can I fill you

   up to survive
is to name everything you own

if it hurts name it
       beautiful

pain flowers in my back

all night all over
a beautiful boy exists

his breath filling me
  up to name him

beautiful beautiful boy

tell me anything

for Will

sit down who you love and tell them
and tell them everything I promise
nothing changes after except sometimes the phone
doesn't ring when you shift your whole self
over it over and over I count
things that won't open again
literally make a list
the names that mouths belong to
the types of fist
my hands around the soft bits of my most difficult body
naked in that summer's bedroom the violence
I am holding was put in my lap
   was taken

Acknowledgements

Thank you to the Troubadour prize for first publishing 'tomorrow my brother died', and to Proletarian Poetry for publishing 'young man,'.

With thanks to all the poets who've inspired and supported me, and a special thanks to all the members of Wayne's Saturday group, Arji, Emma, Iulia, Nick and Tina. To the Poetry School, for building a genuine and supportive community of poets.

A huge thanks to Abi Palmer for her kind words and encouragement, and to Wayne Holloway-Smith for believing in my work, and helping me find my way into contemporary poetry. Wayne is a champion of so many great young poets, and I'm really proud he reckons I might be one of them.

Lastly to Amy and Jake, who've been so supportive, encouraging and kind during this whole process. Writing this book had a big impact on my personal life, and my confidence, and you guys gave me the support and time I needed to come out with something I'm really proud of. Thank you.

New and recent titles from Bad Betty Press

Sylvanian Family
Summer Young

At the Speed of Dark
Gabriel Àkámọ

poems for my FBI agent
Charlotte Geater

The Body You're In
Phoebe Wagner

*And They Are Covered
in Gold Light*
Amy Acre

She Too Is a Sailor
Antonia Jade King

While I Yet Live
Gboyega Odubanjo

The Death of a Clown
Tom Bland

Animal Experiments
Anja Konig

War Dove
Troy Cabida

bloodthirsty for marriage
Susannah Dickey

No Weakeners
Tim Wells

Alter Egos
Edited by Amy Acre
and Jake Wild Hall

Blank
Jake Wild Hall

Raft
Anne Gill

The Dizziness of Freedom
Edited by Amy Acre
and Jake Wild Hall

Forthcoming in 2020

A Terrible Thing
Gita Ralleigh

Field Notes on Survival
Edited by Amy Acre
and Jake Wild Hall

Lightning Source UK Ltd.
Milton Keynes UK
UKHW011338060121
376530UK00002B/676

9 781913 268107